IT'S EASY

Here are t   w
to get you off

Within my   )f
modern, appِ   e
reacted positively to the 'Hay Diet', some with amazing results.

However, we did find some difficulty in applying the diet at first, often getting it wrong. I frequently wished that condensed information was available, especially when away from home. Hence this handbag-sized pocketbook for quick reference. **All the key facts are here.**

I would recommend reading from the many books available on the subject for medical and dietary explanations in depth, and for case histories and recipes.

I wish you luck with my version of the 'Hay Diet food combining' system. The joy of being free from pain, the renewed vitality and the absence of tiredness make the effort well worth while.

Good health!

CHRISTINE RICHMOND
Llanfihangel, 1993

CONTENTS

Our Modern Diseases

Diseases which 'food combining' (the 'Hay Diet' system) can help to cure, control or, quite simply, avoid altogether:

- ALL arthritic and rheumatic pain
- Diverticulitis
- Constipation
- Bloating, ulcers, and other digestive problems
- Headaches and migraine
- Asthma, hay fever, sinus, catarrh and chest problems
- Weight problems and eating disorders
- Skin diseases — from dry, poor skin to eczema, athlete's foot and psoriasis
- Colds and 'flu
- Urinary tract and sex organ disorders — thrush and cystitis
- Diabetes
- Dental decay and gum diseases
- PMT, period pain and irregular bleeding
- Tiredness, mood swings
- Mental disorders
  …and probably much else.

The Diet Explained

THE BASIC DIET CONSISTS OF —

ONE *STARCH*

ONE *PROTEIN*

and ONE *ALKALI-FORMING*

MEAL A DAY

THE AIM IS TO SEPARATE FOODS WHICH REQUIRE DIFFERENT ENZYMES FOR THEIR DIGESTION.

THIS MEANS KEEPING PROTEINS AND FRUITS *APART* FROM STARCHES.

SOME FOODS ARE *NEUTRAL* AND MAY BE EATEN WITH EITHER PROTEINS OR STARCHES

The Alkali-forming foods

- **POTATOES**, especially in their jackets.
- **FRUITS**, including bananas.
- **DRIED FRUITS**.
- **VEGETABLES**, green and root.
- **SALADS** and **HERBS**.
- **NUTS**, almonds, brazils and hazelnuts.
- **MILLET**.

Some foods are alkali-forming, some are acid-forming.

Alkali-forming foods <u>should provide about 80% of our diet</u>. Some alkali-forming foods are STARCH, some PROTEIN, and some are NEUTRAL, so they will be scattered among your starch and protein meals. Consider this when you look at what is on your plate.

<u>One pure-alkali-forming meal should be eaten</u>

<u>each day.</u>

Breakfast is the easiest meal to do this, but it may be taken later in the day.

NB Yoghurt, wheatgerm, butter, and oil may be added to alkali-forming meals.

RECOMMENDATIONS

ALKALI -forming	**_Breakfast_** ↓ *minimum* **2^1/$_2$-hour gap** before next meal	Lemon tea/Ceylon tea. Fresh, squeezed orange juice. Fresh fruits sliced with one tables[wheatgerm and yoghurt.
	Mid-morning *if needed*	Ceylon tea/herb tea/fresh coffee sugar). Oatcake or rice cake.
STARCH meal	**_Lunch_** ↓ *minimum* **4-hour gap** before next meal	Jacket potatoes with butter & seasor Huge mixed raw salad/vegetables. Dressings. Seeds, nuts, dates, figs etc. Bananas, maple syrup, yoghurt/crea
	Tea *if needed*	Ceylon tea/herb tea (no sugar). Fruit (with yoghurt)
PROTEIN meal	**_Supper_** ↓ *minimum* **4-hour gap**	Wine (<u>dry</u>) if liked. Fruit juice. Soup (<u>no</u> potato), or Grapefruit. Fish/meat/poultry/game/eggs/chees 3 or 4 lightly-cooked green/root ve <u>not</u> potatoes. Gravy/sauces. Fruit/fruit salad (<u>no</u> bananas) & cr Nuts.

ALTERNATIVES

things to remember...

- KEEP PROTEIN AND FRUIT IN **SEPARATE MEALS** FROM STARCHES

- Bananas are a STARCH

- Potatoes are a STARCH

- All other vegetables and salads are NEUTRAL — can be eaten with starch or protein meals.

- Eat lots at each meal. I *mean LOTS!*

- KEEP THE GAP between meals for digestion. This is VITAL.

- You may exchange the lunch and supper meals <u>but</u> remember to exchange the mid-morning with the tea as well (if you take them).

- Nuts are fine, but <u>not</u> peanuts!

- Limit tea/coffee to three cups a day, or less.

baked dried apricots.

ɔups (no protein).
ıce/pasta/bread.
at/rice cakes.
ɔrridge. Popcorn.
vocado.
ery sweet grapes.

ıneral waters.
vocado, shellfish.

alad.

aked apple with
isins. Yoghurt/cream.

THE HAY DIET CHART

Protein ———	Neutral ———	Starch
All meats	**Note**	Potatoes
Fish	Neutral foods may	Sweet potatoes
Shellfish	be eaten with	Jerusalem artichoke
Poultry	protein *OR* starch	Pumpkin
Game		
Eggs	ALL VEGETABLES	Bananas, dates, figs,
Cheese	*except*	currants, sultanas
Milk	the 'potato group'	raisins (and grapes,
Yoghurt	(see under Starch)	pears and paw-paw
		— only if *very* sweet)
	ALL SALADS, including	
	avocado, sprouted	
	legumes & seeds	
All fresh FRUIT	Herbs and spices	Cereals
	Butter & cream	Grain, rice etc
	Cream cheese	Pasta

Dried beans, dried peas, lentils etc. (use sparingly)	and sesame oils Egg yolk Nuts (<u>not</u> peanuts) Seeds & raisins Wheatgerm, bran, oatgerm	Oatmeal Milk & yoghurt (use sparingly)
Dry wines & dry cider	Whisky & gin	Beer & ale

Sugar substitutes Maple syrup, a little honey or honey water, concentrated apple juice, orange juice, raisins.

Salad dressings Oil, lemon, mustard, salt & pepper.
Oil & garlic, salt & pepper.
Oil, cider vinegar, garlic, mustard, salt & pepper.
Home-made mayonnaise & cream dressings.
Soy sauce.

Shopping List

Don't start 'food combining' until you have stocked up on the basics. Also, start when you have at least the first week free from 'food social' situations!

- Fresh fruit, veg and salads
- Potatoes, preferably unsprayed, baking, organic
- Garlic
- Yoghurt, plain, the type containing lactobacillus acidophilus — creamy or low-fat
- Butter and fresh cream
- Wheatgerm
- 'Extra Virgin' olive oil, cider vinegar, Dijon mustard
- Herbs, preferably fresh
- Sun-dried fruit — apricots, dates, raisins etc
- Oat and rice cakes
- Bread — preferably wholewheat organic or the delicious yeast-free 'Manna' bread
- Home made wholewheat soda bread (excellent and easy to make)
- Wholemeal flour, oatmeal
- Whole grain brown rice
- Pasta
- Maple syrup
- Nuts — especially almonds
- Bones for stock (make some good sauces!)

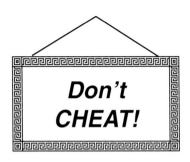

Don't CHEAT!

If you cheat, it can't work! If you stick to the diet, especially in the early stages, the results start to be felt in a matter of days — by day 5 in my own case.

So, give it a fair chance, make sure you have bought in the necessary foods, and plan one day ahead.

Eating Out

I found this difficult at first, especially before I had got the foods and drink sorted into sections in my head. Here are some pointers —

- <u>Dinner & Lunch Parties and Restaurants</u>

Usually easiest to stick to a protein meal and simply leave aside or don't help yourself to bread and potatoes. Choose fruit puds, or cheese.

- <u>Lunch when Shopping</u>

Probably starch is easiest — soups, rolls, jacket potatoes, wholemeal scones, pasta and veg. sauce or salads.

- <u>The Village Hall</u>

If asked to contribute snacks, make sandwiches of cress and walnut, banana and date, or cream cheese and chives. Little biscuits with egg yolk and mayonnaise topped with nuts, peppers, cress etc. Then you can eat from your own offering.

- <u>Air Travel</u>

Take a few apples and a packet of oat cakes to supplement the 'packaged' meals served. Drink mineral water.

- <u>Packed Lunches & Picnics</u>

Soups are a good standby, hot or cold — starch OR protein, then

EITHER —

* Sandwiches or rolls filled with a selection chosen from bananas, dates, nuts, egg yolk, cream cheese, tomatoes, salads etc.

A nut, seed and raisin mix to finish.

OR —

* Cold chicken, meats, prawns, with a mixed salad.

Fruit and nuts.

Special Hints

- Don't inflict your diet on others. Your health and vitality are the advertisement.

- Always check with your doctor before embarking on any change of diet.

- Lightly-cook or steam vegetables until just crisp. You can cook several types together — briefly.

- Raw foods retain their vitamins. Don't boil them away!

- Sugar (especially hidden sugars in manufactured, tinned and packaged foods) is our *NUMBER ONE MENACE!* Cut it down relentlessly.

- Refined flour and cereals are an equal *MENACE.*

- *REMEMBER* — Many of those drugs you take have side-effects. Wouldn't it be good to do without them?

- Soups — A veg. soup (without potato or pasta) may be eaten with either a starch or a protein meal.

- Two alkali-forming meals a day will speed up results considerably. Base one on fruit and the other on potatoes.

- Children, athletes, and those doing much manual work may need extra starch meals.

Allergy?
The Immune System

Many people suffer from allergies — to pollen, oranges, coffee, wheat, milk, and many more.

It is interesting to note that, once established on the 'Hay Diet' food-combining system, former allergies are often no longer a problem. In other words, the immune system is working.

Excessive yeasts are another common modern problem, large amounts being found in bought bread, biscuits and cakes. Cut them, and the sugars they feed on, out of your diet and the results are quickly felt. Thrush, cystitis, bloating and skin diseases are often the result of excessive yeast.

My Mother

My Mother was 80 this year. A few months ago she was suffering from a terrible rheumatic pain in her hip, talking of a hip replacement and feeling generally miserable. Pain makes you miserable.

Now, after two months' of 'food combining', the pain is negligible, she is steadily reducing her anti-inflammatory pills and she is very bright, active and cheerful — and fully mobile, too.

When installing a shower recently, her builder, on learning her age said, "Never! I told my wife you were about sixtyfive!" That really made her day.